THE ONE MEAL A DAY DIET QUICK START GUIDE

Effortlessly Transform Your Body Into A Fat-Burning Machine With OMAD Intermittent Fasting

Landry Kane

CONTENTS

DISCLAIMER

The information provided in this book is designed to provide helpful information on the subjects discussed. This book is not meant to be used, nor should it be used, to diagnose or treat any medical condition. For diagnosis or treatment of any medical problem, consult your own physician. The publisher and author are not responsible for any specific health needs that may require medical supervision and are not liable for any damages or negative consequences from any treatment, action, application or preparation, to any person reading or following the information in this book. References are provided for informational purposes only and do not constitute endorsement of any websites or other sources. Readers should be aware that the websites listed in this book may change.

Intermittent fasting is safe for many people, but it's not for everyone. Skipping meals may not be the best way to manage your weight if you're pregnant or breast-feeding. If you have kidney stones, gastro-esophageal reflux, diabetes or other medical problems, talk with your doctor before starting intermittent fasting.

If you enjoy this book and feel like you can benefit from the information provided, would you please leave me a quick review when you're done? I would truly appreciate it and you will be helping others find this information as well.

I read every review and I would love to hear your feedback!

You can leave at review at: bit.ly/OMADDIET

Thank you!

Sincerely,
Landry Kane

INTRODUCTION: HOW WOULD IT FEEL TO BE FREE?

How many diets have you been on in your life? Have you lost count? Do you beat yourself up when you fall off an eating plan? How many times have you told yourself *"this time* it will be different"? Believe me, I completely understand. I've battled with my weight since I was a child. Up until a few years ago, I felt trapped in a cycle of starting a new diet; telling myself that I'd stick with it this time; falling off the plan; being mad at myself; eating more; gaining the weight back; being convinced I had to do something about my weight; finding out about a new diet ... and then I'd start the cycle over again. Can you relate to this?

You might feel like I did at that time. I felt desperate to change – but after countless attempts (with only short-lived positive results), my cycle of failure left me feeling hopeless that things could ever change permanently.

What if you could trade in that hopeless feeling for

an expectation that you can and will succeed? And not just short-term success, but a lasting total body and health transformation?

How would it feel to be free? Free from doubts; free from failure; free from disappointment and free from the all-too-familiar diet restrictions? Sounds pretty incredible, right?

At this point, you might be a bit skeptical. *Every* diet book on the market tells us "*This* is the answer you've been looking for!" So, I can understand your hesitation. I felt exactly the same way before I discovered intermittent fasting. How could this be different than any other approach to weight loss?

I was burnt out on dieting. I didn't want to try again. I thought if every diet eventually ended in disaster, why should I bother trying anymore?

Around that time, a friend of mine discovered intermittent fasting and was raving about it. Although it sounded interesting, initially I wouldn't even consider it as an option because I wasn't interested in going on another diet.

When I saw the results that my friend was getting, I was amazed. The extra pounds seemed to melt off of her and she radiated with confidence. Even though my walls were up, I started to do more research on the topic. I read a few books on intermittent fasting and was blown away. Could it be true that there was a way that I could successfully and sustainably reach my fat-loss goals? I had my doubts. But it sounded so different from everything else I've tried over the years. I realized I had another try in me.

I started practicing intermittent fasting and was fascinated at how the pounds seemed to effortlessly come off. Where had this way of eating been all my life?

It ends up that it's been around much longer than me (I am 50 years old) but it had fallen out of popularity in recent years. This is mainly due to the fact that modern society (in general) has lost sight of the immense benefits of "less". We've turned into a people always desiring "more".

In recent years, the idea of "less" has been increasing in popularity again. With concepts such as minimalism, decluttering and downsizing becoming more mainstream, we are starting to embrace the same ideas around our eating behaviors. Do we consume meals and snacks all day long because we should? Or because it's what our culture finds acceptable? Is it simply a habit? It's time to question what we think we know. Especially if the ideas we've been hanging onto haven't been serving us. I didn't even question my old view of requiring several meals a day. I thought it was a fact - it turns out that it is not.

I have tried (and enjoyed) many different types of intermittent fasting. I'll cover some of the different ways to practice it in Chapter 1. But my favorite has always been the One Meal A Day approach. Instead of restricting the amount of food (number of calories) or types of foods (i.e. no carbs or no fat), it simply restricts the time that you eat the foods you choose. There are no other limitations! This is a liberating discovery. You can eat the foods you desire (with no restriction on the amount) at a certain time of day. That's it! There are no other diet rules to remember. You can finally be truly free.

This book is designed as a quick-start guide that will get you going on your One Meal A Day plan as soon as possible. It's packed with all the basics to launch your successful journey.

I'm thrilled for the opportunity to pass along the information that has helped me to escape the diet/weight-gain cycle. I hope you're excited as well.

If you're still hesitant, that's ok. Just keep reading. I hope and pray that you will discover what I did – there actually is a different way! One that is simple and one that *works* for the long-haul. Now let's jump in to the fun!

CHAPTER 1: WHAT IS OMAD?

Let's start with the basics. Fasting simply means: willingly abstaining from food (or calorie-containing beverages) for a specified amount of time. There are many different ways that people practice intermittent fasting (sometimes referred to as "IF"). There is no one "right" way to go about it. Some popular examples of different ways to practice fasting are:

16:8 Fasting

The person will refrain from eating or drinking calorie-containing beverages for 16 hours every day. They consume all their food in an 8-hour period.

20:4 Fasting (Sometimes Called The Warrior Diet)

The person following this plan will refrain from eating for 20 hours every day. They consume all their food in a 4-hour period.

5:2 Fasting

Just when you thought you had the number pattern figured out, I'm throwing 5:2 into the mix! 5:2 fasting indicates that the person will eat "normally" for 5 days out of the week and will abstain from food for 2 days a week. Typically, the fasting days are not consecutive. An example of this would be going without food every Tuesday and Thursday – but eating regularly the other 5 days out of the week.

Alternate Day Fasting

A person following an alternative-day fasting regimen would eat "normally" on one day and fast for the next day. Additionally, some people add in one 500-calorie meal on their fast days while following this plan.

There are countless ways to observe intermittent fasting. These are just a few examples. The main aspect that they all have in common is that it is a pattern or rhythm of eating. To establish this rhythm, the person who is fasting will typically eat their food during the same time-period every day. This is also known as an "eating window".

An example of this would be someone following a 20:4 fasting schedule eating their food between the hours of 4 and 8 p.m. every day. Therefore, that person's daily "eating window" would be 4 p.m. – 8 p.m.

Please note: there is definitely room for flexibility and special occasions when you are following an intermittent fasting routine. But it is most beneficial to stay within a relatively consistent eating window to gain the most benefit from your fasts.

Here it is. The one you've been waiting for! The One Meal A Day Diet is also known by its acronym O.M.A.D. (or simply OMAD).

In my opinion, the One Meal A Day Diet is superior to all other ways of practicing fasting because you'll be enjoying the benefits of a maximum daily fasting time (allowing you to lose more weight or lose at a faster rate) while also allowing you to eat every day.

Plus, when you eat, you'll be able to eat whatever you want with (almost) no restrictions on the amount of food you can have! I say "almost" because everyone is different. One person may be able to eat unlimited portions and dessert every day, and another might need to limit that to a couple of times a week. We'll discuss this more in Chapter 4.

The bottom line is that you will no longer have to count calories …or carbs …or fat grams, etc. For the most part, you can eat what you want, in the amounts that you desire. How freeing would that be? You won't have to worry about what you "can" or "can't" have. You can simply enjoy yourself and your food. When friends or family invite you out, you won't have to choose between them and going off your diet. You can finally eat like a non-dieting person, while seeing amazing weight-loss results! Does this sound too good to be true? It's not.

People are rediscovering the incredible benefits of the ancient art of fasting. This is no fad. There is a reason why it's gaining momentum and popularity – because it WORKS.

OMAD is also sometimes referred to as 23:1 – meaning, you consume all of your food for the day within one hour. If only eating in a one-hour time period sounds impossible, I assure you it's not. You're most likely drawing off of experiences you've had in the past. Who hasn't skipped a meal, only to be ravenous later in the day? Because you've lived it before, you can't imagine feeling that same restriction (and subsequent "I-want-to-eat-everything-in-sight" feeling) day after day. Hang in there. Don't give up now. I promise you that it will not feel like that every day.

There are many factors that add up to the negative feelings and reactions we've had in the past after skipping one or more meals. Some of them are biological and some are habitual. We'll get deeper into that in the next chapter. For now, please just trust me when I say that once you get used to your new routine, you won't believe how easy it is to skip the other meals you used to eat.

It's best to keep this hour at approximately the same time every day. So, if it's important to you to eat dinner with your family, have your OMAD meal between 5 p.m. – 6 p.m. If your job requires you to take lunch or breakfast meetings, it would make more sense to choose an earlier time of day.

Although there has been much discussion and debate within the diet and weight loss community over what the best time of day to eat is – my opinion is there is no "correct" time. The time of day that is best to eat is the one that YOU can consistently stick with. In the past, I've eaten my one meal at dinner. More recently, I've switched it to mid-day. I find that only having to wait till lunch is easier for me during the day. When I have a filling meal that sustains me (which is the goal), by the time I'm starting to feel a bit hungry again, it's time to go to bed.

I want to stress that this is personal preference. Once you get used to eating one daily meal, you can try different times of the day and see what works best for you. I don't suggest playing with the times too early into your journey. Consistency in the beginning will help you more easily adjust to your new plan.

In the next chapter, we'll uncover the benefits of intermittent fasting. Not only can it help you lose weight easily and safely, but it can also transform your health and your outlook on life. Let's get to the good stuff…

CHAPTER 2: THE AMAZING BENEFITS OF INTERMITTENT FASTING

Intermittent fasting not only can turn your body into a fat-burning machine, but it also has countless health benefits. Plus, it can save you money and actually give you more time in your day to do the things you need to accomplish (or have always wanted to do)!

Fasting Benefits

According to intermittent fasting expert, Dr. Jason Fung, just a few of the health benefits derived from fasting are as follows:

- Weight/fat loss
- Lowering of blood insulin and blood sugar levels
- Increased energy
- Improved blood cholesterol levels
- Improved mental clarity
- Increased cellular cleansing, due to autophagy

- Increased growth hormone
- Reduced inflammation
- Possible reversal of type 2 diabetes

Although most of the benefits included in the list above are self-explanatory, there are a few that might not seem that exciting at first glance. Let's take a deeper look at a couple of them.

Autophagy

The word autophagy was derived from the Greek meaning "eating of self". At first glance, that doesn't sound like a good thing... until we take a closer look. It actually means that after fasting for a certain amount of time, our body "eats" the weak/damaged cells for energy and recycles them to make new, healthy cells. This is extremely important because when autophagy is activated, it gets rid of the bad cells that have the potential to cause serious diseases down the line.

According to lifeapps.io, autophagy is an important process for cellular and tissue rejuvenation – it removes damaged cellular components including misfolded proteins. When your cells can't or don't initiate autophagy, bad things happen, including neurodegenerative diseases, which seem to come about as a result of the reduced autophagy that occurs during aging. Within 24 hours, (of fasting) your cells are increasingly recycling old components and breaking down misfolded proteins linked to Alzheimer's and other diseases.

Wow! Possible increased protection from neurogenerative diseases while achieving your weight-loss goals sound pretty awesome to me!

Reduced Inflammation

According to npr.org, inflammation can be a force for good, protecting against infection and injury. Acute inflammation occurs when you sprain your ankle or get a paper cut. It's part of the immune system's box of tricks to spark a defense and promote healing. But when that response is constantly triggered, over time it can damage the body instead of healing it. Chronic, low-level inflammation seems to play a role in a host of diseases, including type 2 diabetes, heart disease, Alzheimer's, cancer and even depression.

According to the Mayo Clinic, research suggests that intermittent fasting may be more beneficial than other diets for reducing inflammation and improving conditions associated with inflammation, such as:

- Alzheimer's disease
- Arthritis
- Asthma
- Multiple sclerosis
- Stroke

Reducing inflammation in our bodies is a must if we want to live long, healthy and vibrant lives. As opposed to a regular intermittent fasting routine, simply eating less does not have the same results in reducing inflammation.

In addition to all of the benefits that we've covered, medical professionals believe that there are countless more that we haven't discovered yet. With more research being conducted on intermittent fasting, science is constantly discovering more ways that it is beneficial to our bodies.

Weight Loss Benefits

In addition, the act of simply reducing fat and returning your body to a healthy weight carries many benefits with it, such as: decreased risk of diabetes; lowered blood pressure; improved cholesterol levels; decreased risk of heart disease; decreased risk of certain cancers; decreased risk of stroke; reduced back pain; decreased risk of osteoarthritis; decreased risk of developing sleep apnea; greater confidence; improved sex life; better sleep; elevated energy levels; decreased stress and better mood.

Saving Time and Money

It might sound crazy at first – but you will actually save time and money when you follow the One Meal A Day Diet!

Think about it – if you are only consuming one meal every day, it will save you time in the following areas:

- Deciding what you'll eat or drink
- Preparing the meals (or picking them up)
- Time spent consuming the meal
- Clean-up time afterwards

I understand this doesn't apply to everyone. Many of you, like me, still have to prepare food for your families. But for those who it does apply to, this will be a game-changer.

It might not sound like a lot of time, but it quickly adds up. If you didn't have to take all the steps listed above twice a day, you'll definitely have more time to dedicate to other things you'd like to accomplish. Even using a conservative estimate, you'll gain at least an hour back every single day. What could you do with an extra hour every day?

Another added bonus is that you'll save money when you follow this plan. For those of you with families that are still consuming the traditional three meals a day, this might not be evident right away. For those who only prepare your own meals (or for you and one other person), the difference will be substantial. This not only applies to the money you'll save at the grocery store, but you'll also save on dining out, take-out, snacks, etc.

Mental & Emotional Benefits

I personally believe that this is one of the most exciting changes that you'll experience. The difference that you'll see in your mental and emotional states will be mind-blowing. You won't have to talk yourself into feeling better – it will happen automatically and naturally. Two of my favorite benefits in this area are as follows:

You'll gain more self-confidence.

Not only because you're getting closer to your fat-loss goal, but because you'll be proving to yourself that you CAN be successful in this area of life. When we experience countless diet failures, it's easy to adopt an underlying attitude that conveys "I can't really do this." The doubt is always there. But when you start making strides and realize you can do it, your confidence will soar. An added benefit to this is that you'll start to notice this confidence spreading to other areas of your life.

You'll be free from a diet mindset.

When you no longer hold the mindset that you "can't have" certain foods or can only have a small amount, everything will change! When "forbidden" foods don't exist, it takes away all of their power. Personally, this was the single most powerful change in my mindset when I switched to intermittent fasting. After feeling like I was in a prison for countless years, I was finally free. The restrictions were gone and I could truly enjoy food once again without feeling guilty.

Fast and easy weight loss; transformed health; extra

time and money; mental clarity and freedom? Sounds good to me! I hope you're getting excited. OMAD really is all these things and more.

Next, we'll have a look at what is happening inside the body to make this way of eating so simple and powerful. Let's move on to Chapter 3…

CHAPTER 3: WHAT'S HAPPENING INSIDE MY BODY? THE ONE THING YOU NEED TO KNOW.

If you have an interest in discovering exactly what is happening inside the body when you practice intermittent fasting, there are countless resources available. Because 1) this is a quick-start guide and 2) I am not a doctor, I am going to boil this down to the single most important thing you should know about what is happening inside your body when you fast ...or when you break a fast.

On the other side of the coin, if you have absolutely no interest in the science behind what makes OMAD so powerful, I still believe that it is extremely important to know **WHY** you shouldn't have "just one bite" of pizza or "that one sip" of a delicious latte during your fasting hours. That *one* tiny bite or sip will set into motion metabolic processes that can throw off your entire fast.

Because there aren't many rules on OMAD, the ones

that are in place *must* be followed to the letter. The first rule of OMAD is don't talk about OMAD. Just kidding. The first rule is to only consume foods and calorie-containing beverages during your eating window. Eating anything outside of that time will discount your fast and make it much less powerful.

If I'm having a weak moment or feeling hungry, I usually ask myself, "is it really worth a bite?" The answer is usually no. Again, there are times to be flexible such as family gatherings, being out with friends, a wedding or other celebrations, etc. But when it's a bite of a donut in the break room at work – skip it! You'll be happy you did. Here's why...

What Happens When We Eat? Extremely-Simplified Edition

When a relatively healthy person consumes calories (from food or a beverage), their blood sugar rises. The body responds by releasing insulin, the main hormone responsible for energy storage. Insulin takes the energy that has just been consumed and ushers it to the places it needs to go inside the body. Some of the energy is used immediately and some is saved for later use. A limited amount of this energy can be saved as sugar. This gives the body quick-access to energy for the near future. But once that limited short-term storage is filled, the body goes to work storing the rest as fat.

Insulin is our friend because 1) it takes the energy we've eaten and ushers it to the tissues and other areas of our bodies that need it, and 2) it helps to lower our circulating blood sugar levels, since it can be dangerous if they remain elevated. That being said, insulin can also be a friend that turns on us if we don't treat him well.

Listen up. Here's your main take-away for this chapter: **when insulin is present in the bloodstream, your body locks up your fat storage-units. No stored fat can be burned as long as insulin is present.**

That's it? Yep. That's it.

Well, of course that isn't really the entire story. Our bodies, which have been created in a miraculous fashion, go to work taking care of the countless processes that need to occur to keep us going. But, as far as what you need to take away from this chapter, that is it.

You only need to remember that insulin in the bloodstream interrupts your fast – no matter how small the amount of food. Again, it doesn't matter if it's one M&M or one sip of juice. The end result is that your body will release insulin. That is what we want to avoid during our fasting hours.

There is some controversy in the fasting community about whether weight loss comes about because there is a cap on the calories that can be consumed in a short period of time. Some people are convinced that this is just another way of restricting calories. Because I am not a medical professional, I cannot definitively answer that question. My opinion is that weight loss comes about as a combination of both. I believe that giving the body a chance to let the insulin levels drop (and therefore, make it easier to release fat from storage) in conjunction with an overall slight reduction in calories creates the perfect combination and the best environment for easy weight loss. From my experience, it is my opinion that 2/3 of the weight loss power in fasting comes from the decreased insulin levels and that 1/3 can be attributed to natural (not forced) calorie restriction.

According to dietdoctor.com, the body only really exists in two states – the fed state and the fasted state. Either we are storing food energy (insulin is in the bloodstream and we are increasing fat stores), or we are burning stored energy (no insulin is in the bloodstream and we are burning our fat stores).

When we eat from the time we get up till the time we go to bed, we never give our bodies the chance to be in fat-burning mode. This can only happen when we give it a complete rest, in the absence of any food or drinks that contain calories.

Our bodies are so used to being in the fed state, that we constantly need more to keep our energy up. Once you start giving your body the chance to rest and regularly enter the fasted state, you'll find that your body will be happy burning the stored fat.

When your body is in the fasted state, you'll find that you'll typically experience very little hunger. There is one caveat to this: you have to give your body the chance to adjust. Don't expect this adjustment to happen overnight. But it WILL happen. You will be amazed at how little hunger you'll experience during your fasts once your body adapts.

The reason you've felt ravenous after skipping a meal or two in the past is because your body wasn't used to entering the fasted state. This will quickly change. Plus, knowing that a beautiful and completely satisfying meal is coming soon will help you through hungry times in your adjustment period.

I hope this helps you to understand a fraction of what is going on inside your body when you're practicing intermittent fasting. If you want to know more, you can find countless resources online. For now, just remember this: insulin in your bloodstream = no fat burning. It's not worth the bite.

I'd like to give a small disclaimer and remind you that what is described above is what typically goes on inside a relatively healthy body. If you have diabetes, other health issues, or if you are on any medications (especially medications that regulate blood sugar), your body is most likely not responding in this way. It is extremely important to discuss this with your doctor and get their approval before embarking on this, or any other type of new eating regimen.

Next we'll dive in to every dieter's favorite questions: "What can I eat?" and "How much can I eat?" Join me in the next chapter!

CHAPTER 4: HOW MUCH CAN I EAT & WHAT CAN I EAT?

When it comes to learning about a new eating plan, these are the questions that every dieter wants to know the answers to:

- How much am I allowed to eat? And,
- What can I eat on this plan?

The amazing news is that when you practice The One Meal A Day Diet plan, there are almost no restrictions on how much you are able to eat or what you can eat and still lose fat.

That being said, OMAD is **NOT** a license to binge once a day. As with everything, there is a balance.

Because every person is different, you'll need to discover what works for you and what doesn't. I wish I was able to give you clear-cut instructions in this section. But there is no one-size-fits-all approach. And isn't that really the beauty of it? You have the opportunity to design a plan that works for YOU. No one will be telling you what you can or can't consume. This is a wonderful thing because you can tailor the OMAD plan to your personal needs/preferences.

First, let's take a closer look at the amount of food you'll be consuming.

How Much Can I Eat?

The short answer is that you can have as much food as it takes for you to feel satisfied. Of course, this is not the entire answer.

Before we get into a few more details on this subject, I want to encourage you that you will not have to think too much about this. If you're new to fasting, your internal panic alarms might be sounding right about now. "What if I get so hungry that I eat everything in sight?" or "I won't be able to control myself!" I promise you, that within a couple of weeks, this will cease to be one of your worries. It might sound completely foreign right now, but once you are used to this new rhythm of eating, you will not want to eat as much as you have in the past. That's right. And this is coming from a former binge-eater!

I don't have the scientific reason behind this phenomenon – but I do know that it takes a much smaller amount of food for me to feel full. Give yourself some time to adjust. The first 2-3 weeks might not reflect this. But be kind to yourself. Expect that it will take some time to fully adjust and for your hunger to dissipate (more on hunger later).

I wanted to start with that encouragement to save you from worrying about managing the amount of food that you will eat when fasting. OMAD is a way of eating that will *free* you from all of the over-thinking and micro-managing of food. Your body will tell you when it is done eating. You'll have to be patient with yourself in this area too. It will take some time to re-learn what the correct amount is for you.

I have spent many times feeling stuffed and overly-full after my OMAD meal. Other times, I tried to restrict myself (which was a mistake), and I'd feel hunger sooner than I'd like to. As you start to pay attention and become more in-tune with your "feeling full" cues, this will be easier to navigate.

Another factor that plays in to how much you'll be able to consume and still lose fat is your current weight. When I started, I needed to lose almost 100 pounds (about 45 kilos). Obviously, someone needing to lose 20 pounds (about 9 kilos) would not be able to consume the same amount of food as I could at that point. Although you'll have to do a bit of self-discovery and see what works for you, (again) I don't want you to get too hung up on this, because I honestly believe it will become obvious and self-regulating – even for those who have a history of extremely poor eating behaviors, like I did.

What Can I Eat?

Again, the short answer is: you *can* eat anything that you would like (during your eating window). But because everyone has different likes/dislikes, sensitivities, allergies, preferences, cultures, etc. What you choose to consume will vary from person to person.

That being said, my suggestion is to start your meal with wholesome foods in their natural state. Some examples of these types of foods are non-processed meats, fish, eggs, nuts, seeds, fruits, vegetables, etc. If you choose to abstain from consuming meat, starting with a protein source will serve you well.

The reason it is best to begin your meal with these types of foods is that they offer much more nutritional value than processed foods. For your body to perform at the optimum level and for you to feel good, you need these nutrients! Plus, it is easier to get them in at the beginning of the meal. The odds are that you won't squeeze them in at the end. Then you can move on to any treats or desserts that you'd like to incorporate.

For example, I usually eat my foods in this order: meat, salad or vegetable and then bread and/or dessert. I save my treats until later in the meal, since I'm less likely to overeat on meat or salad.

When I'm ready for my treat, I enjoy it freely. *No guilt allowed.* Please do the same. My hope for you is that you will learn to fully and thoroughly enjoy your food once again. Instead of carrying around guilt over what you "should" or "shouldn't" eat, you can re-learn a good relationship with food. The best part is that this will come naturally over time. You won't have to force it.

As I briefly mentioned in the last chapter, although calories do play a role in your weight loss, you don't have to be overly concerned with them… and *please do not* start counting calories (unless you enjoy that type of torture). OMAD is designed to free you from the shackles that have held you back in the past. Simply eat in your "eating window"; give it some time and everything else will fall into place. That being said, if you have a very small amount of weight to lose, you might not be able to eat as much as you'd like to. Although I still wouldn't suggest counting calories, you might want to limit treats and/or breads to a few times a week, instead of having them every day. Follow what your body is telling you.

What Can I Consume During My Fast?

In order to set yourself up to have the most success with The One Meal A Day Diet, you should only consume the following during a fast:

- Water (filtered or sparkling, no additives). Add lemon, if desired.
- Black coffee
- Unsweetened tea

That's it. That might seem scary at first glance. But if you think of all the amazing benefits that IF can provide: the easy weight loss and being able to eat almost anything you want during your eating window – this is totally worth it!

If you're wavering, review Chapter 3 and remember that **insulin in the bloodstream = no fat being released**. Drink some water, tea or coffee and tell yourself that your next delicious meal is right around the corner.

Next we'll cover how to get started with OMAD and how you can choose to ease in or jump in like a cannonball. Join me in the next chapter.

CHAPTER 5: GETTING STARTED WITH THE ONE MEAL A DAY DIET

Like everything in life, there are varying opinions on the best way to start intermittent fasting, especially the OMAD plan. I will once again tell you that there is no "right" way, so you should do what is most comfortable to you.

Some people ease into the practice and others simply jump right in. I am a "let's-jump-in" type of person. So when I started, I simply decided on an eating window and one day I restricted myself to only eating during that time and I didn't stop.

If that sounds crazy and scary to you, no worries. You can ease into it. Here are a couple of suggestions on how you can do that.

Skip A Meal

Does only skipping breakfast sound less intimidating? Or perhaps eating breakfast and lunch while skipping dinner sounds better to you. Either way, pick a meal and start regularly skipping it. The key is consistency. The more you do it, the more your body will get used to this new eating pattern. Once you're used to it, you only have to skip one more meal to get to OMAD.

You can stay with skipping one meal for days, weeks or months. Whatever it takes for you to feel comfortable moving to the next level.

Shrinking Your Eating Window

Let's say you are currently eating from 7:00 a.m. when you have breakfast until you have a snack at around 9:00 p.m. That means that you are currently eating in a 14-hour eating window. You can start by shrinking your eating window by an hour per week (or whatever rate is comfortable for you). You'll keep shrinking the window until you achieve the 23:1 OMAD window.

Tip: Once you reach a 4-hour eating window, you're basically already where you need to be. It's hard to fit in more than one truly large/satisfying meal in less than 4 hours. As I sit writing this, I ate my OMAD meal 3 hours ago and I still feel comfortably full. Plus, you'll be sleeping 6-8 hours a night, which will take up a large part of the fast. You'll get there sooner than you think you can.

You WILL Experience Hunger

I wish I could say that you won't. But you will experience hunger. I want you to be prepared ahead of time, so you will have realistic expectations. In our culture we're not used to being hungry. We typically grab something to quench it as soon as it arises.

The good news is that it *will lessen* over time. It is usually the most pronounced in the first week or so while your body is adjusting. As time goes on, you will feel less and less hunger. There are days that I feel no hunger whatsoever. This is a typical response in people who practice IF. That being said, there are days that I do still feel hungry. Here are a few tips that can help you overcome the hungry times:

- Drink water, tea or black coffee.
- Remember that hunger comes in waves. Just wait it out. It might seem overwhelming… and then it will simply disappear.
- Do something to distract yourself (work, play, etc.)
- Tell yourself that your next wonderful meal is just around the corner. It's worth the wait.
- Change what hunger means to you. Instead of it signifying lack or deprivation, tell yourself that you are BURNING FAT from your fat stores.

Losing weight (especially if you've carried extra weight for a long time) can be a battle in the mind even more than a physical battle. If we can make these simple changes in our thinking, it can completely transform our outlook on the process. If we get stuck thinking thoughts such as: "Poor me! I'm deprived. Look at what my family is eating. I want some. This isn't fair!" it's easy to ride that slippery slope down to a bad place. But if we start reminding ourselves that soon we'll be able to enjoy a delicious and satisfying meal, while the fat falls off... it will be easier to stick to only eating in our eating window.

Instead of thinking "I *have to* stay on my plan." switch it to "I *get to* follow a simple plan in which I can eat whatever I desire until I'm satisfied, while losing fat! How awesome is that?"

If you eat outside of your window, be kind to yourself. Just get right back on. We all go off plan sometimes. But the good news is that is extremely easy to get back on the OMAD plan. Most dieters, including me in the past, tend to have an "the diet starts Monday" attitude. Once we fall off, we eat everything in sight until it's time to "get back on". With OMAD, there are no forbidden foods, so it takes this destructive attitude out of the equation. So what if you ate in a 4-hour window one day? Just get back to your 1-hour window tomorrow. Easy. You'll be pleasantly surprised at how easy it is to eat (and be successful) in this way. I can't wait for you to discover this for yourself.

CHAPTER 6: DO I HAVE TO EXERCISE TO HAVE SUCCESS?

You may be asking, "do I have to exercise in order to have success with OMAD?" Once again, I'll give you a short version of the answer as well as a longer explanation.

The short answer is no. You do not have to work out in order to see amazing fat loss results with OMAD. That being said, there are countless benefits that are associated with exercising and being active. Therefore, I highly encourage you to have some activity in your day (if you don't already).

It seems as though many people have a negative attitude towards exercise. I think this is derived from a collective attitude of "I *should* be more active." It's that "*should*" that makes it sound like a chore, so we interpret and internalize it in that manner. But what if we looked at being active in a new light? Remember back to when you were a child. Most children love to run around, ride their bikes, play sports, skateboard, play with pets, play tag, you name it! As we get older, it turns into a "should" rather than a "I get to". As a kid, you'd think "I get to play outside!" as an adult, we think "I have to exercise".

What if we could get a bit of that enjoyment back into our lives? Try taking a walk, playing a sport you used to enjoy or biking around the park. Try to switch this back to being an "I get to" activity.

Any of these activities can be fun and done at a leisurely pace. As a society it seems that we've made everything *extreme.* The "go big or go home" mentality has driven many of us to stay home! When it's a fun and enjoyable activity rather than an extreme energy-drain, it becomes something that we can look forward to, instead of something we can't stand doing. Anything we dislike doing will not be sustainable in the long run. That's the bottom line.

One last encouragement to you regarding exercise... when your body is in the fasted state, the only place it can pull energy from is your fat stores! Therefore, when you do any activity in the fasted state, it burns the fat right off your body. Instead of having to burn through the sugar in your bloodstream and "short-term" storage areas, it targets the stubborn fat you've been storing on your body. If that isn't motivation to get out and move, I don't know what is!

If you've enjoyed this book and feel like you've benefited from the information, would you please leave me a quick review? I would truly appreciate it and you will be helping others find this information as well. I read every review and I would love to hear your feedback!

You can leave at review at: bit.ly/OMADDIET

CONCLUSION & THANK YOU

Thank you so much for letting me lead you through this quick-start guide of The One Meal A Day Diet! I hope that you're excited to get started. I wish you all the success in the world. I pray that you will discover and claim all of these amazing benefits in your own life. Don't let this information simply remain as words on a page - get out there and give it a try! It might be challenging at first. But if you make it through 2 days, you've made it through the hardest part. Don't give up! Keep going. Because it will only get easier from there. I can't wait for you to see the results for yourself.

If you've enjoyed this book and feel like you've benefited from the information, would you please leave me a quick review? I would truly appreciate it! I read every review and I would love to hear your feedback!

You can leave at review at: bit.ly/OMADDIET

Now get out there and change your body and life!

Sincerely,

Landry

REFERENCES

Fung, M.D., J. F. (2020, July 18). *Intermittent fasting for beginners*. Diet Doctor. dietdoctor.com/intermittent-fasting

JARREAU, PHD, P. J. (2020, May 18). *THE 5 STAGES OF INTERMITTENT FASTING*. Life Apps. lifeapps.io/fasting/the-5-stages-of-intermittent-fasting/

HOBSON, K. H. (2017, July 21). *Is Inflammation Bad For You Or Good For You?* NPR. npr.org/sections/health-shots/2017/07/21/538377221/is-inflammation-bad-for-you-or-good-for-you

Mundi, M.D., M. M. (2020, April 21). *What is intermittent fasting? Does it have health benefits?* Mayo Clinic. mayoclinic.org/healthy-lifestyle/nutrition-and-healthy-eating/expert-answers/intermittent-fasting/faq-20441303